Anorexia

A Parent's Guide - How to Help Your Child Overcome Anorexia

By Lynn Johnson

Mirror
Mirror
on the
Wall,
Who's
the
Thinnest
of
Them
All?

Disclaimer

If you or a loved one needs screening or diagnoses, please seek out professional evaluation. Because denial is often part of the disorder, seeking medical evaluation may come only at the insistence of a family member or close friend.

This book contains only general information and should not replace professional medical and psychiatric treatment.

This book contains the opinions and ideas of its author. It is intended to provide useful information on the subject matter covered. It is sold with the understanding that the author is not engaged in rendering professional services in the book. If the reader requires professional assistance, a competent professional should be consulted.

The author specifically disclaim any responsibility for any liability, loss, or risk, personal or otherwise, which is incurred as a consequence, directly or indirectly, of the use and application of any of the contents of the book.

Dedication

This book is dedicated to my mother, father and brother (Stewart Johnson Sr., Diane Johnson and Stewart Johnson Jr., who spent hours and hours crying, fretting and caring for me. They are an amazing family, without their encouragement, I might not have survived anorexia.

Acknowledgments

 I would like to my husbands family. Diana Meyer, Fred Meyer and Daniel Michalski, have raised such a wonderful son.

I am also thankful for my best friend, Jill Anderson. She has also been a major support throughout my life. She is truly extraordinary. We have been friends since the age of 5 and will remain friends forever.

Table of Contents

Preface

This book is a true story of how I became anorexic at age eleven and of how after many years of treatment - I learned to manage this horribly deadly disorder. Now, at age 39, I live a healthy and wonderful life with my husband and three wonderful children.

It was almost impossible to treat my anorexia because I
- Didn't believe I was underweight
- Didn't want to be helped
- Thought I looked fat
- Thought people were secretly trying to
    "fatten me up"
- Obsessed constantly about my weight
- Worked out to the point of exhaustion

This book can help any parent who has an anorexic child to overcome these obstacles and become a healthy and productive member of society.

If you or a loved one needs screening or diagnosis, please seek out a professional evaluation. Because denial is often a part of the disorder, seeking medical evaluation may come only at the insistence of a family member.

This book contains only general information and advice about eating disorders and should not replace professional medical and psychiatric treatment.

Chapter 1
My Story

I grew up in a suburb of Milwaukee, Wisconsin. My family was "somewhat" normal. I had a brother named Stewart Jr., a mom and a dad. My brother was really good at biking and skating. My parents worked in the fine arts.

We lived in an average house and had a dog named Poochie. Well, Poochie ran away all the time. About once a week we had to chase him in the car - with hotdogs dangling out the window - yelling "Pooooochiiiiieeee". After many chases, finally my dad said he took Poocchie to a farm where animals lived happily ever after. I believed him, well sort of. Then we got a cat named Mittens. He was a nice black cat with white paws. He never tried to run away but did like to bring dead mice home in his mouth.

A lot of the kids that I went to school with were extremely rich. I'm talking really, really rich. Most of their parents were doctors or lawyers.

One of my friends named Joanne, whose dad was a lawyer, had a "maids house" in her front yard that was as big as our house. They even had a trampoline, a swimming pool and a tennis court. I used to go over to her house and play. I would get jealous because her closet was so huge compared to mine.

Another friend, Michelle, lived right by Lake Michigan. She had the most beautiful red brick house. It was so big that we used to practice gymnastics in the front hallway. We also loved to play hide and seek

because there were endless "great hiding spots".
Michelle got new clothes every single week. She was so
spoiled. Was I jealous? Yes, of course. We had a very
nice house, but it was not a mansion.

I guess it all started, my obsession with food and
weight, when I was about 9 years old. I had a good
friend, named Amy, who was pretty, popular and yes -
very thin. I also had another friend, Suzy, who was also
extremely pretty, popular and yes, thin. *These two girls
were not very good influences on my self-esteem.*
I actually had a best friend named Jill. She was a
very good friend to me. *We met at age 5 and have been
friends ever since.* We had so much fun together as
children. We performed puppet shows for the
neighborhood, had lemonade stands and we laughed
about everything. Jill's mom, would say we had
"gigglitous" because we couldn't stop laughing.
Sometimes we laughed so hard, we peed in our pants.
Then, we laughed about peeing in our pants.
Jill was a major boost to my self-esteem. She
seemed to bring out the best in me. We loved to laugh
and share stories. We always cared for each other. She
was an excellent swimmer and had a fantastic muscular
body.

Although I was never overweight, I was not thin
either. I was average for my height - but compared to
my two friends - Amy and Suzy- I thought I was fat. I
thought I was not as cute, nor as popular as they were.
I thought I was just average - plain and boring.

I thought if I became thin, I would be invited to every single birthday party, dance and friends house.

When I would go over to Amy's house after school to play, Suzy would come over and the three of us would play games like - stuffed animals and dress up. We would try on Amy's older sister's clothes and pretend that we were teenagers. I was never very excited to "dress up" like a teenager. In fact, I did not want to become a teenager at all. I did not want "big breasts." Because I thought any breasts were "fat". I thought if I had breasts I would look like a cow. In fact, I did not even want hips.
I just wanted to be straight and thin like Amy and Suzy.

Whenever Amy's Mom came home after work, she would serve us a snack. She always offered me more food (than Amy or Suzy) - saying that I was bigger and probably needed more food. This stuck with me for a long time. I thought, maybe she thinks I'm fat - she must, if she says I'm "bigger.

Funny thing - at age 30 -I learned Amy's mom had bulimia. Amy had also been extremely bulimic as a teenager and college student. She did recover as a young adult.

I began ballet classes at age 6. Every Saturday my mom would drive us girls to ballet class. I really loved learning to dance. But I always compared myself to Amy - she was thin, I was average. She was gracious and beautiful - an excellent dancer -always in the front of the line when we did leaps across the floor. She was extraordinary. I was not.

Strangely enough, - at age 16 - I became a superb dancer - not a ballet dancer - but a Jazz and Modern dancer. I was in a dance company and performed many solo dances. I even had a full tuition scholarship. Its strange how things work out.

At age 11, I started to develop - this really freaked me out. My mom took me to get a bra. I thought everyone could tell I had bra on at school. It was so embarrassing. The boys would snap on your bra when you weren't looking. I didn't really like wearing a bra. Then, my periods started, I didn't really think that was too fun either. *Now please, don't worry my story does have a happy ending.*

My obsession with my weight started in gym class. Our gym teacher would weigh everyone in the springtime. I did not like being weighed on the scale. Afterwards, all the girls in the locker room would compare their weights. Even at age, 11, they talked about how much they weighed and if they looked fat in the mirror. I became a scale watcher, a mirror watcher and a people watcher. I constantly compared myself to other girls - especially Amy and Suzy.

My mom was always on a diet. She was somewhat overweight and wanted to be slim. One time, I asked her why she was overweight...she said it was because couldn't take the weight off after the pregnancies. This really freaked me out. I thought, I would never ever get pregnant. I would never ever get fat.

Every day after school I would weigh myself, not once, not twice, but 10 times at least. At 5'2" tall, I was about 90 pounds. I thought this was way too much. Amy only weighed 80 pounds. Suzy only weighed 85 pounds. I thought I was fat. I started to cut back on "fatty foods."

During lunch I would only eat half of what my mom packed. I started losing weight. Within a few weeks, I was about 78 pounds. I felt in control of my weight. I felt powerful. It was the only thing in my life that I really did have control over. ***Many anorexics girls feel "in control" of their eating. Especially when things in life seem "out of control", for example a divorce or a move to a new school, losing weight can be thought of as the only thing the anorexic patient can control.***

Everyone at school seemed to notice I was losing weight. They said - wow- you look so skinny. I took it as a complement. I loved all the attention. Every time someone commented on my weight - I thought - I must look really good.

Soon, my periods stopped, which to me, was a good thing. I didn't really like that "bloody mess" anyway.

At age 12, I tried out for cheerleading. I made the team. Amy, of course, was captain. She said I could be her assistant. That sounded great. Cheerleading was fun except for the locker room talk. All the girls talked about was dieting and how fat they looked in the mirror. *Anorexia typically appears during adolescence, about one to two percent of the female population between the ages of twelve and eighteen if affected.*

At some point, I decided that 78 pounds was too fat. I decided to go on another diet. This time I wanted to be 68 pounds. I stopped eating altogether. I dropped more weight, and yes - got the attention I craved. Teachers, classmates and my parents noticed. To me, it was good attention. I was thin and noticed by everyone at school. To me, it was great to be thin.

I obsessed constantly about food and weight. Mealtimes became stressful. I didn't eat much, only very low calorie foods. I started to hide my food in my napkin. I felt very guilty about eating anything that I thought would make me fat. I memorized a calorie counter book. I would only eat really low calorie foods.

(But really, I didn't feel good. I was depressed, lonely and very tired all the time. I was at a very low point. Cheerleading practice even seemed too hard. I was cold all the time.)

I didn't really feel hungry. Just really scared of food and mealtime. I counted every single calorie and obsessed constantly about food.

I actually liked cooking and making meals for other people in my family. I would cook great food, but then not eat very much.

One day, I got sick - really sick. My mom took me to the doctor. He said I had bronchitis and needed medication.

He weighed me at the office and was shocked that

I was only 72 pounds. Even though the doctor said I was "OK", my mom knew I had a problem and took me for evaluation at a psychiatric hospital.

Parents need to trust their own instincts, not necessarily trust all doctors. Second opinions are very important.

FIRST HOSPITALIZATION

The next day, my parents took me to the hospital. I did not really agree to this idea. *I did not think I needed help.*

I did not want any help. Somehow, they managed to get me admitted. It was the scariest day of my life.

I started out in a very small unit. Unit 3. I t had only 5 or so patients, most of them were "way out of here." One boy had schizophrenia, one had tried to commit suicide, another was an alcoholic and one girl was skinny. They said she had an eating disorder - anorexia - but to me, she looked good. Her name was Becky. *She was even thinner than me.* She never smiled and barely talked. She was not very friendly. She had to be watched constantly because she would throw up her food. She couldn't even go to the bathroom by herself. She also would try to exercise in her room. She had to keep the door open at all times and be monitored in the bathroom.

As a side note - I think Becky did finally recover and lead a pretty normal life.

The first day, my psychiatrist Dr. Machi stopped by. He didn't say much. But told me I would be gaining weight. He said my goal weight would be 100. *I hated him! He would not make me gain even a pound! I cried.*

I yelled. I said I wanted to go home. He said I would be given privileges (like talking on the phone or watching television) only if I ate 3 meals and 2 snacks daily and gained 5 pounds. I would be given 3500 calories a day, until I gained up to 100. Then, he said, I would go home.

I did not want to gain weight. *But I did want to go home and be skinny again. I wanted to go back to my old ways.*

My thirteenth birthday was the next day. I was very homesick. My birthday was horrible. I was lonely and forced to eat food. I was not allowed any visitors because I was in Unit 3. It was the worst birthday ever.

I really wanted to get out of Unit 3. I had a plan. I would get to 100 pounds and then go home and go back on a really super strict diet until I reached my goal again of 68 pounds.

I was a terrible patient, because I did not want treatment. I did not want to gain weight. I did not want help! Due to the disorder, I ended up missing 5 months of school.

What would have helped, maybe, would have been to teach me about "healthy choices" and "Healthy body image" and "the dangers of being so thin".

I fought the doctors and nurses constantly about eating. I would sit at the table with Becky and the three other patients and refuse to eat. Usually Becky would beat me out. She sat at the table at least 2 hours per meal. Taking only very tiny bites. She tried to hide her food in her pockets. They caught her. She obviously did not want to go home.

Unit 3 was so small and so boring. The only person to talk to was the nurse, Becky or the other three "way out there" patients. Becky told me she wanted to go home also.

Dr. Machi said when I gained 10 pounds then I would move to Unit 2 and have a roommate. He did not come to the Unit 3 very much. Maybe two times a week just to stop by and say hi. I refused to talk to him except to tell him - I WANT TO GO HOME NOW.

Dr. Machi told me I would be in Unit 3 until I gained 10 pounds - or about 82.

I could not believe it. I thought I had been tricked!!! I only weighed 72 pounds and looked great or so I thought.
Really, I looked terrible, I had huge bags under my eyes and my bones stuck out of my shoulders and hips. It even hurt to sit - because my butt was so skinny. My face looked very old and saggy.

Becky looked very thin to me, but she was also my competition. She would sit at the table, and refuse to eat. She had to sit there until she finished her plate, which took her several hours at each meal.

I finally gave up fighting about food and weight and just ate to "get out of the hospital."

Finally, I was allowed to go to Unit 2 and get a roommate. Her name was Nicole. She was in the hospital for suicide. She said I should gain a few pounds because, "Boys don't like skinny butt girls. She was really funny. She made me laugh. *Once I reached about 90 pounds, I started to get back my sense of humor and energetic personality. This was a good sign.*

But, I was not out of the closet yet.

I was allowed to go home for a three hour pass. On the visit, I refused to eat and exercised for about an hour in my room. *When my parents said it was time to go back to the hospital, I fought - really fought - kicking, yelling and punching them.* Trying to stay home, I cried the whole way back to the hospital. I hated that doctor and hospital. *They actually had to call a security guard to strap me in a binder and take me back to the unit where I was stripped nude and checked for laxatives, knives, etc. I hated the strip searches. I was not allowed to go home for another 4 weeks, due to bad behavior. I thought this was very unfair.*

One day, Dr. Machi said I would be going to a group session with other anorexics. Well, it was a group session - but not much talking. Most of the anorexics were quiet, sullen and very thin. *Group therapy did not work for me, because I learned more anorexic tricks to losing weight - like extreme exercise, binging/purging and use of laxatives, hiding food, wearing baggy clothes, etc. Looking back, I would say these sessions actually made me worse because I would compare myself to the other anorexics and think...I am so fat!*

Finally, after five months of hospitalization and missing school, I was allowed to go home. I had reached my goal of 100 pounds. I did not like the way I looked and was ready to start dieting right away. **Obviously, I was not at all cured.**

I went right back into my old ways. Quickly, I lost weight. Within a few months I was 85 pounds but I didn't want my parents to know. I would hide under baggy clothes and started binging and purging. Binging on food really upset me. I did not like to be out of control. After a starvation of 4 days or so, I would have a giant binge, and then use laxatives. I felt horrible and embarrassed to tell anyone about binging. The binge/purge cycle was very difficult to treat and I needed hospitalization once again.

My parents noticed I was thin, and took me back to Dr. Machi. I actually put ankle weights and lots of stuff in my pockets so I would weigh more. Dr. Machi noticed and was very mad that I had lied. I was immediately hospitalized.

When I was sick and in the hospital, I isolated myself from friends and family. I was so embarrassed to have a "problem."

SECOND HOSPITALIZATION

This time, I was admitted at about 84 pounds. I was very depressed and lonely. But, I was a little more open to treatment. I started to talk to my doctor and we started family therapy with Dr. Perry Johnston. He helped our family understand the disorder and made me realize how much commotion I had created. My brother had been ignored because I was sick. I felt guilty for taking up all their time and attention. I felt sad for not being "normal" and *I realized that I needed to try to solve my eating disorder.*

During the second hospitalization, I opened up and really tried to understand anorexia/bulimia. I wanted to be normal, but I still thought I was fat.

As I gained weight and reached my goal of 100 pounds, I actually became more stable emotionally and admitted that I had a problem. *Just because I admitted it, however, did not mean I was free from anorexic tendencies and behaviors.*

I celebrated my 14th birthday, again in the hospital. It was pretty sad.

I was only hospitalized for 4 months the second time. When finally allowed to go home, I was in a pretty good space and ready to start my Junior Year of High School. Boys were of interest and my weight was pretty stable. I found a boyfriend and started to drive. I loved dancing and became a great dancer. Somehow, I managed to maintain a weight of about 95-100 pounds.

SELF-MANAGEMENT OF ANOREXIA

I graduated from High School and went College to obtain and degree in Psychology. Then I got a Masters Degree in Advertising and Marketing. I was very self-disciplined and an excellent student. I became obsessed with my professional success and studied to the point of exhaustion. You could say I was obsessed with my professional life.

Secretely, I still wanted to help myself get better. I was not cured. I knew my obsessive/compulsive behavior was exhibiting itself in my work. I was actually pretty stable and did not want to be severely underweight. I maintained about 95 pounds by eating healthy and exercising daily.

In college, I met my future husband, Mark. *He has been the greatest support for me. He is so intelligent and understanding. He always encouraged me to "solve it myself."*

After dating for a few years, we got married.

Then, I got my Masters Degree in Advertising and he got his MBA. I worked in advertising and was actually pretty stable, maintaining about 95 pounds for many years. *But really never quite cured from anorexic or obsessive behaviors.* I worked really hard at my job. I was obsessed with my job as a sales representative. I wanted to be the best. I was the best. I won trips and awards.

Then one day, I decided I was on the wrong path. I knew I was too stressed out as a sales rep. I wanted a major change. So I said, "Honey, let's move to Hawaii."

We had a little money and so we decided to sell our house, sell all of our stuff and move. It was very exciting to plan a new life in Hawaii.

Hawaii was even better than we both imagined. We loved the ocean, the mountains and the sky. It was magical to live there.

We were very lucky to get jobs right away. My husband worked in the financial field and I worked in advertising doing graphic design.

Hawaii was a great place to live. But, we were far away from our families and support systems. I think this may have contributed to my relapse into the world of anorexia once again.

RELAPSE

A about age 26, one day I started to cut back on food. I stopped eating meat. I started exercising more, sometimes, three or four hours a day. I lost weight. I did not think I was losing weight because I did not really weigh myself. *I did not think I had a problem.* But my clothes did feel baggy and my face seemed to sag again.

My husband and mother said I looked too thin. I thought they were lying. *I was in total denial. Once again, I did not want help. I did not want to change my behavior. I was scared to eat certain foods and terrified of eating out at a restaurant.*

I suffered for the next two years with severe anorexia and no help. I was very malnourished. People stared. They thought I had Aids. I had severe depression and mood swings. I was not very emotionally stable.

At age 28, I hadn't had a period in about 2 years, and went to the OB doctor. I thought maybe I was pregnant. I was shocked when the doctor said I only weighed 78 pounds. I did not believe her or her scale. She told me I needed to gain weight because she was concerned I would end up with osteoporosis. I didn't even know what osteoporosis was.

She said my periods stopped because my hormones were at the level of a ten year old girls. I needed to be a normal weight or else I would be crippled with osteoporosis at a very young age.

She explained that my heart was a muscle and that my body would start to eat itself if I did not gain weight. She told me I could have a heart attack at any time and I needed to gain weight immediately. *For some reason, I believed her. I knew she had my best interest in her words and in her heart.*

I was more scared of osteoporosis than of being fat. I wanted help, but at times I didn't want help.

The doctor also prescribed Prozac. She said it would help with my moods. I decided to try it and it did actually seem to make me feel better. *I think that Prozac actually was a lifesaver. The medicine helped me to stop thinking obsessively about food and stabilized my moods. It was actually amazing to feel happy again.*

BREAKTHROUGH

I also started to imagine what I would look like at a healthy weight. *But, I was scared to gain the weight.* I was terrified to eat "real food."

At that point, I couldn't even walk because my leg and feet muscles had deteriorated to nothing and I had no energy. My feet really hurt. It was as if my feet muscles were being eaten by the anorexia. I had pain when walking. My hands were orange and my face was orange from eating too many carrots. Also, I had severe stomach pain and couldn't tolerate milk products. *I was in really bad shape and should have been hospitalized.*

My mother tried to intervene, but as an adult couldn't really hospitalize me that easily. ***My husband said I needed to solve the problem on my own. He told me I could do it.*** He had incredible faith that I could beat the disorder head-on.

I knew I had to change my eating or else I would die. I knew I had to change my way of thinking or else I would die. **I knew I was headed in the wrong direction and I had to turn it around.**

I struggled with my own self-talk. I tried to change the way I thought about food (instead of food as the enemy, food as my fuel for living). I read many health books and started making really healthy well-balanced meals.

For the first time in my life, I really wanted to get over the anorexia for good. I really wanted to be healthy and live a long life. I knew if I didn't change, I would end up dead.

But, changing my thoughts was not so easy. I went to see a fitness instructor. He helped me envision a new body - with new muscles.

I started to visualize myself as strong muscular and athletic. Because I was so weak, the only form of exercise I could do was swim. Slowly, I started to train for a mini Ironman triathlon. I swam, biked or ran each day - with my goal of completing the mini triathlon. I even started lifting weights.

As I gained weight, I gained strength both physically and mentally. I became stronger and was noticing a change in my physique. I thought - WOW - I am looking like a super fitness model. My husband encouraged me and even made the best grilled hamburgers for me to eat.

I ate alot of protein - like protein shakes, hamburgers and even steak. *For some reason, I didn't feel guilty eating the protein - I thought of it as fuel for my muscles.* I even started taking vitamins and supplements daily.

Over time, I gained muscle, not fat, and looked incredibly strong, much stronger than I had ever been in my whole life. I loved the way my legs and arms looked - lean and strong. I eventually got back to about 95 pounds. My periods returned and I looked really like a woman - but a very athletic woman. I felt really good about having gained muscle and reaching a healthier weight for my petite 5'2" frame.

After about 6 months of solid training, I was ready for my mini Ironman. I ran 6 miles, biked 20 and swam ½ mile in the ocean in Kona, Hawaii. I completed it with ease and was very proud of myself to have reached my personal goals of healing my anorexia mentally and physically. My period even returned to a somewhat normal cycle. I couldn't believe it. I loved my new body and was very thankful for having had the support and faith of a wonderful husband.

BABY TIME

Then one day, at age 29, my husband said he wanted to have children. I WAS TERRIFIED. I DIDN'T EVEN KNOW IF I COULD HAVE CHILDREN. Had I ruined my whole body? Had I destroyed my own ability to conceive? How could I possibly gain 25 pounds to maintain a healthy baby? How could I do that after just recovering from anorexia? *My husband knew I could handle it and gently encouraged us to begin a family.*

Miraculously, I got pregnant immediately. I was so amazed and excited. I had a normal pregnancy and delivery. I lost the baby weight and was around 100 pounds within 8 weeks. I was amazed at the whole process of having children and how natural it seemed. I didn't feel fat when I was pregnant. I just felt pregnant. *For anyone reading this who has been anorexic and recovered, it is possible to have children. However, it is necessary to be at healthy weight when conceiving.*

After the first child, we moved back to Wisconsin to be closer to our family. This was actually a hard transition, because I loved Hawaii and really did not want to leave the beautiful Big Island.

I wanted more kids, so I had two more children. They have been the most amazing additions to my life. I know I must take good care of myself, both physically and emotionally, so that I can set a good example for my children. I eat a well balanced diet, exercise regularly, and maintain a healthy weight.

Now, at age 39, I have 3 healthy kids - 2 boys and 1 girl. **It is now even more important for me to maintain my health and set a good example for my children, especially my daughter.** I want to make sure that she has a healthy and positive self-image and grows into a healthy woman. I take good care of myself and continue to exercise and maintain a healthy weight. **I try to be a good role model for my children.**

FULL RECOVERY

I can say now, that after many years of suffering, I am finally able to manage this horrible disorder - anorexia. I know that an anorexic lifestyle and behaviors are unhealthy and self-destructive.

I am extremely happy that I have a caring and supportive husband who believed in me and in my own ability to solve my problems.

Chapter 2
What is An Eating Disorder?

Definition of Anorexia Nervosa

The clinical definition for diagnosing anorexia nervosa is that the individual maintains a body weight that is below a minimally normal level for age and height. The threshold is less than 15% below normal weight. The following is a diagnosis criteria for Anorexia Nervosa:

DIAGNOSIS CRITERIA FOR ANOREXIA NERVOSA

A.   Refusal to maintain body weight at or above a minimally normal weight for age and height (weight loss leading to maintenance of body weight less than 85 percent of that expected; or failure to make expected weight gain during period of growth, leading to body weight less than 85% of that expected).

B.   Intense fear of gaining weight or becoming fat, even though underweight.

C.   Disturbance in the way in

which one's body weight or shape is experienced, undue influence of body weight or shape on self evaluation, or denial of the seriousness of the current low body weight.

D. In postmenarcheal females, amenorrhea, i.e., the absence of at least three consecutive menstral cycles. (A woman is considered to have amenorrhea if her periods occur only following hormone administration, e.g. estrogen.

SPECIFIC TYPES

Restricting Type: during the current episode of anorexia nervosa, the person has not regularly engaged in binge-eating or purging behavior (i.e.-self induced vomiting or the misuse of laxatives, diuretics, or enemas).

Binge-Eating/Purging Type: during the current episode of anorexia nervosa, the person has regularly engaged in binge-eating or purging behavior (for example, self induced vomiting or the misuse of laxatives, diuretics, or enemas).

Signs and Symptoms of Eating Disorders (Anorexia Nervosa, Bulimia Nervosa and Binge-Eating Disorder)

The signs and symptoms of eating disorders vary with the particular type of eating disorder.

- **Anorexia Nervosa.** Essentially self-starvation, this disorder involves refusal to maintain a minimally healthy body weight, and in severe cases, anorexia can be life threatening.
- **Bulimia Nervosa**. This disorder involves repeated episodes of binge eating followed by weighs to purge the food from the body or prevent expected weight gain. People can have this condition and be of normal weight.
- **Binge Eating Disorder**. This involves frequent episodes of overeating without purging.

It is important to note that there are varying degrees of severity with each disorder. For example, one anorexic may be in a very severe and life threatening state and require immediate hospitalization while other anorexics may be able to receive care and recover as an outpatient.

In the past, eating disorders were thought to start during the teen and young adult years. Now researchers, clinicians and mental-health professionals are saying they're seeing the age of their youngest anorexia nervosa patients decline to 9 from 13 years old.

Recent studies have shown, eating disorders are not only starting earlier, but there is a surprising diversity among patients. Not only are anorexic patients more likely to be black, Hispanic or Asian, they are also more likely to be boys, more likely to be middle aged - all of which goes against the conventional wisdom that victims are mostly white, type A girls from privileged backgrounds succumbing to pressures. This means that parents and teachers have a responsibility to monitor their child's dietary habits and be aware of any negative changes.

Anorexic Signs and Symptoms

- Weight loss, sometimes achieved by self-induced vomiting, abuse of laxatives, use of diuretics or exercise.
- Refusal to maintain a normal body weight, sometimes weighing 15 percent or more below normal body weight
- Acute anxiety of gaining weight
- Obsession with food
- Negatively altered body image
- In females, menstrual changes or the absence of menstruation.
- Ritualistic behavior at mealtimes
- Fatigue, depression, dizziness
- Drying and yellowing of the skin
- Irregular heart rate
- Baby fine hair covering the body
- Mild or severe anemia
- Brittle nails and hair

Bulimic Signs and Symptoms
- Recurrent episodes of binge eating
- Feeling that you can't control your eating behavior
- Eating much more food in a binge episode than in a normal meal or snack
- Following a binge with efforts to prevent weight gain - such as self induced vomiting, using laxatives or other medications, fasting or excessive exercise
- Often performing binge/purge behavior in "secret"
- Unhealthy focus on your body shape and weight
- Dehydration
- Fatigue, depression, dizziness
- Constipation
- Damaged teeth and gums from gastric acid contained in vomit
- Swollen cheeks from regular vomiting
- Irregular heartbeat

Binge-Eating Disorder

- Recurrent episodes of compulsive overeating not followed by purging
- No control over eating behavior
- Feelings of guilt or shame
- Fatigue, depression
- Joint pain
- Gallbladder disease
- Increased blood pressure and cholesterol levels

Causes of Anorexia

The causes of anorexia are not certain. It appears a variety of factors contribute including genetics, family behavior and culture. In some instances, researchers have found the biological systems in the brain that govern appetite and digestion are not functioning properly.

New research is offering clues about the causes of anorexia. Recent studies have shown that the levels of serotonin activity in the brains of anorexics is abnormally high. These pumped up levels of hormone may be linked to feeling of anxiety and obsessional thinking, classic traits of anorexia. Studies have shown that anorexics may use starvation as a mode of self medication.

Some researchers suspect genetics plays a role in the likelihood of a person developing the disorder. It appears there is an increased risk of anorexia nervosa among first-degree biological relative of individuals with the disorder. One study of anorexic women indicated two percent of patients' sisters and mothers also had the disorder. Other research suggests this rate of anorexia among first degree relatives may be even higher.

Some psychiatrists see family situations as possible contributors to mental disorders. One theory is that families of anorexics have strict and rigid expectations. In such situations children find it difficult to meet the challenges facing teenage years.

In addition, the messages sent by the media that excessive thinness is attractive contribute to the cause of anorexia. To be as thin as some teen models would require people to achieve a weight that's not healthy.

Everywhere you look there are messages that being fat is bad and dieting is the solution. Young children are very vulnerable to these messages and sometimes take them literally.

Sam, for example, thought if he ate anything with "fat", he would become fat. This irrational belief lead to dieting, excessive weight loss and finally an eating disorder.

Randy saw an advertisement for a diet pill and assumed that she must need a diet pill. She started dieting and couldn't stop. Eventually the diet pills caused heart palpitations and extreme nervousness.

Although many advertisements are targeted towards overweight people, everyone is repeatedly exposed to them. This repeated exposure can be detrimental and lead to irrational beliefs about food and weight. Especially for young girls and teenagers there is an overwhelming amount of messages sent regarding dieting and weight.

America's obsession with food and weight can be seen in Seventeen and Cosmopolitan magazines. Yet, most of us are not born with bodies that will ever look like the models in magazines. No matter how hard we try, we can't make one body type into another. Billions of dollars are spent each year on advertising showing very thin models. This often leads females think they are fat, and go on a diet. At times, dieting becomes so severe that it leads to nutritional deficiencies and eating disorders.

Risk Factors

Studies have shown that risk factors include gender, age, family influences, heredity, and emotional disorders.

The majority of eating disorders occur in teenage girls and women in their early twenties. Those who have close family members with eating disorders and those with other emotional disorders are also at high risk of developing an eating disorder.

Psychological Aspects

ANOREXIA IS A SYMPTOM
OF OTHER PROBLEMS
An eating disorder is not just a problem with food and weight. It is a symptom of underlying problems. For example, an anorexic who has a low self image (feels worthless or unattractive), may focus entirely on the number she sees on the scale as a value of her self worth. The lower the number, the greater her self image becomes - she may feel the number gives her power - I am thin, I am good, etc. The weight is not the real issue, but the self esteem which is closely tied to the weight is. By focusing on weight, exercise and food, an anorexic is able to avoid thinking about other problems (maybe the parents are arguing and she fears they may get divorced).

ANOREXIA AND DEPRESSION
GO HAND IN HAND
Anorexia is often accompanied by depression. In some cases the patient may be "clinically depressed" and have severe depression including loss of interest in life, sad moods, low energy levels, sleep problems.
In some cases the depression may have contributed to the eating disorder, while in other cases the depression may be a bi-product of the eating disorder itself. When a person has an eating disorder, they are not getting proper nutrition and as a result, their brain cannot function optimally leading to internal

chemical imbalances in the brain and dramatically affecting mood and emotional stability.

ANOREXIA IS USED AS A PACIFIER

Some eating disorders patients use food as a pacifier in their life, especially anorexics that have bulimic symptoms as part of their disorder. Binging on food is used as way to deal with problems or feelings that are unresolved in one's life.

For example, Sally, a bulimic, may be upset that she didn't get a job promotion, this may trigger a binge/purge cycle. She may go home from work extremely frustrated and angry and take it out on herself by eating a whole pie and three gallons of ice cream and then throw up. Instead of confronting her feelings of inadequacy in regard to her job, she uses the food as a tool for comforting herself. However, the binge/purge cycle makes her even more upset and depressed. She feels out of control and angry that she let herself eat "all that food". Then she may start to restrict her diet again. After three days of dieting, Sally has another unresolved problem- she thinks her boyfriend is cheating. Sally again uses food as a comfort, instead of dealing with the real issue - her relationship with her boyfriend.

ANOREXIA AND DENIAL

Another interesting facet of anorexia is that anorexics often become defensive and deny insist that nothing is wrong. This makes it a very difficult situation for family and friends. How can you get help for someone who doesn't want help or think they need help? In many cases with children who live at home, an intervention is planned and the patient is forced to get help for their eating disorder. This is sometimes the best option if the patient is in severe physical condition and also in severe denial.

FAMILY ISSUES

Family problems are often a psychological aspect of anorexia. For example, in an unstable household where the parents are on the verge of divorce, a child may stop eating in order to bring their parents back together.

Most cases of anorexia are thought to occur in upper/middle class families that have strict rules and rigid expectations. Many anorexics tend to be perfectionists and very successful in school. The high expectations set by the parents may indeed contribute to their need for perfection - not only in academics but also in their physical appearance. Some anorexics are highly competitive in dance or gymnastics - which often pressures girls to be thin. The anorexic does not want to fail, and is very eager to please. She wants to meet the expectations set forth and may go overboard to be physically perfect. Ironically, once the disorder sets in and the anorexic becomes extremely underweight, their body becomes dangerously malnourished and in need of immediate medical attention.

SELF IMAGE

An anorexic lifestyle is very self-destructive. Once the disorder is in full swing, the anorexic belief system and self-talk changes, to support the lifestyle. Much of the day revolves around issues of food and weight, as seen in the following examples:

Obsesses with food and liquid intake
> Counts calories, keeps charts Measures specific amounts of food

Concerned about weighing too much
> Thinks about weight often
> Checks weight on scale often
> Keeps chart of weight

Tries to control dietary intake
> Very upset if doesn't have control

Exercises compulsively
> (sometimes in secret or at night)
> Often, more than 4 hours a day
> to the point of complete exhaustion
> Works out to maintain low weight

Eats food in ritualistic manner
> Eats at certain table, cuts food up in specific way
> Becomes very upset if routine is interrupted

Thinks irrationally/negatively about self
> Sees oneself as fat in mirror, when actually thin
> Doesn't feel he/she is ever good enough
> Not ever satisfied with the way he/she looks
> Thinks specific body parts are gross and fat, even when severely emaciated
> Becomes isolated- especially around

mealtimes
Secretive about what she is/is not eating
Anxious to eat out in restaurant
Hides food in napkin
Goes to bathroom to purge food
Believes others are trying "fatten her up"
Does not trust others - does not believe they
are really trying to help
Denies there is a problem
Becomes extremely defensive when
confronted by family
Becomes angry when confronted and refuses
to get treatment

Seeking Medical Evaluation

If you or a loved one needs screening or diagnosis, please seek professional evaluation. Because denial is often a part of the disorder, seeking medical evaluation may come only at the insistence of a family member. This book is only to be used as general information about eating disorders and should not replace professional medical and psychiatric treatment.

Complications

There are several short and long term complications of anorexia nervosa, bulimia nervosa and binge eating disorder. These include but are not limited to heart disease, hormonal changes, imbalance of electrolytes and minerals, nerve damage, digestive problems, lowered immune system, low potassium levels, teeth and gum problems and even death. About ten percent of anorexics die. Anorexia is a killer, it has the highest fatality rates of any mental illness, including depression.

The effects of anorexia on the body are horrid. When the body is deprived of food over a long period of time, the body cannibalizes itself for energy, first burning its fat stores, then turning to muscle and eventually its own organs.

The heart is significantly affected by anorexia. Starved of energy, it can't pump properly. Patients feel weak and have trouble keeping warm. Electrolyte shortages can cause heart palpitations. In addition, hypokalemia (potassium deficiency) is a major problem for people with anorexia. Chronic hypokalemia can cause an irregular heartbeat, which can lead to heart failure and death.

The kidneys are also affected by anorexia. A severe lack of fluids can lead to organ failure.

During anorexia, muscle tissues are weakened and muscle atrophy sets in, sapping strength and mass, and often making patients feel exhausted and run-down.

If self-starvation lasts long enough, bones are robbed of essential nutrients like calcium which can lead to many bone fractures, early onset of osteoporosis and a weak skeletal system. Especially, in children, calcium intake is crucial for building the foundation of a strong skeletal system.

Anorexics digestive system is also likely to be negatively affected by self starvation. The GI tract slows, leaving patients feeling constipated and bloated. This can exacerbate their already strong aversion to eating.

Extreme weight loss from anorexia disrupts sex-hormone production. This can delay puberty in boys and girls. Girls who remain anorexic during puberty and into adulthood can suffer from infertility.

In anorexia, protein deficiencies cause the hair and nails to become brittle. Also, the skin dries out and is easily bruised.

The brain's ability to function is also dramatically affected by anorexia. Children and adults can become lightheaded and unable to think straight. Chemical imbalances can occur and lead to feelings of anxiety, depression and obsessional thinking.

Treatment Options

In severe cases of anorexia, the patient will require immediate hospitalization in order to restore electrolyte imbalance and weight gain. Other treatments include psychotherapy, group therapy, nutrition education, medications, and family counseling.

Hospitalization-

In many instances, the anorexic may be treated as an outpatient, living at home but visiting the hospital for regular evaluation and treatment. However, if the doctors feel it is necessary, the anorexic will be hospitalized and treated as an in-patient. This may be the case when an anorexic is severely underweight and requires a feeding tube and bed rest, in order to be sure death does not occur.

If a patient is very ill, they will start out with a feeding tube, then move to a liquid diet. Six balanced meals a day are usually recommended. The doctor may start out at 1500 calories a day and then gradually increase the amount to 3,000 or more calories per day. The staff must keep a watchful eye over the anorexic patient because the patient may try to vomit after a meal. The bathroom is usually off limits after meal times in order to ensure the food is digested. The staff and doctors will monitor the anorexics weight. Usually a patient is expected to gain a quarter of a pound a day.

Hospitalization may last anywhere from 2 months to 6 months to one year. As the patient progresses, a system of rewards or privileges is implemented to allow more freedom. For example, after gaining 10 pounds, the anorexic may be allowed a 3 hour pass to visit family and friends.

Eventually, the patient is released into the real world. This, of course, is the hardest part. It is then up to the family to encourage healthy eating and weight maintenance. As an outpatient, there will be regular visits to ensure management of the disorder.

Many anorexic patients do relapse and require repeated hospitalizations, so it is very important for parents to be aware of the signs and symptoms of eating disorders.

Psychotherapy

Psychotherapy, is often used to treat anorexia. A therapist must first gain the trust of the anorexics. This is often very difficult, due to the nature of the disorder. Most anorexics do not believe they are thin and do not want to be treated. This can be a major obstacle for a therapist to overcome.

It is crucial that the patient fully understand that they have a serious eating disorder, which can have very serious short and long term consequences. The therapist must convince the patient that change is really needed. Most anorexics will be extremely resistant to change and very angry about gaining weight.

Family Therapy

Family therapy can be essential to the treatment of eating disorders. Often there is tension or stress in the homes of these patients. Many issues may be explored and resolved in family therapy.

In many clinics around the country, family

participation in the treatment of anorexics is becoming the trend. Families are encouraged to treat anorexia like a disease, with food as the medicine. The family is trained to become a sympathetic support team, especially during mealtimes. This approach seems to work well with adolescents, but not with adults.

If parents of anorexic have their own mental disorders or addictions, they should go not only to family therapy, but set up their own individual therapy and support system.

My mother was advised by another mother of an anorexic, "If you want to help your child, you must get help for yourself." My mother took her advice and it changed her life for the better.

Group Therapy

Group Therapy or support groups can play a big role in treatment. By sharing experiences and stories with other anorexics, they may realize that they are not alone. This may provide support from others who face similar disorders.

Nutrition Education

Many times, anorexics have lost touch with the real world - of how to eat. They have entered into their own special eating universe - where only certain foods are available to them (in their eyes). They first need to be re-taught how to eat and how to feed themselves without feeling guilty. Nutrition education can be helpful in combination with other treatment methods.

Certain foods may be easier for an anorexic patient to digest. Some foods are both nutritious and high in calories. Peanut butter, nuts, bananas, protein shakes, protein bars and dried fruit are good choices for adding calories without the extra full feeling. Anorexics do not like to feel really stuffed and benefit from eating six small meals a day.

Anorexics should eat a well balanced diet that is high in fiber with plenty of fresh fruits and vegetables. These foods are cleansing to the system. When the body is cleansed, the appetite tends to return to normal. In addition, anorexics should avoid white flour products, processed food, and junk food because they tend to add to the aversion to eating.

Medications

Today, doctors often prescribe antidepressant medications to treat the depression and anxiety that often accompany eating disorders. Usually, doctors prescribe serotonin reuptake inhibors (SSRIs) such as flouxetine (Prozac), sertraline (Zoloft) or paroxetine (Paxil). Other antidepressants prescribed include venlafaxine (Effexor) and imiprmine (Tofranil).

The psychiatrist will usually start the patient out on a small dose and gradually build up to the maintenance dose. The use of antidepressants in children and teenagers is somewhat controversial. Some studies have shown that antidepressants can make teenagers suicidal. Please be aware of the side effects of the medicine prescribed to your child. Sometimes, several medications are tried before finding one that is well tolerated by the patient.

In order for antidepressants to be effective, they must be taken as prescribed. Once the patient is up to the maintenance dosage level, continual monitoring by the psychiatrist is necessary because relapse may occur. The doctor may then need to change the dose or switch to another medication.

All medications should not be suddenly stopped. A doctor needs to work with the patient as medications are decreased or stopped. Parents should also learn the side effects of prescribed medications and what foods and/or drinks should be avoided in combination with the medication. The parent should be sure all the medications the anorexic takes are compatible with each other.

Alternative Therapies

Nutrition therapy is also highly recommended as part of a treatment plan for an eating disorder patient. According to recent studies, the liquid form of zink sulfite is beneficial in the treatment of anorexia and bulimia.

In addition, Vitamin B12, D and E are often low in the blood of eating disorders patients. These vitamins may need to be supplemented.

The following herbs have been shown to stimulate appetite: ginger root and ginseng. These herbs may be especially helpful to the anorexic patients.

It is very important for the parent to research hospitals, specialists and doctors in their region, in order to obtain the best care possible for their child.

Chapter 3
How To Help Your Child

You may be wondering, how can I help my child overcome this disorder?

Based on my personal experience with anorexia, I would give the following advice to parents of anorexics…

Never forget that you are the anorexics most important role model. They need you to set a good example of diet and exercise. If you are constantly dieting, stop dieting. Begin a healthy program with a wide variety of foods. Also, show your child how to take care of their body physically with exercise. Try to exercise on a regular basis with your child.

If you care for yourself and your body, they will admire and respect you more.

Realize that anorexia is very hard to cure and will require you to be consistent with your anorexic child. You will need to give her much more positive attention than usual, and reward her for small healthy changes in eating/weight. Remember, eating and gaining weight usually makes an anorexic extremely anxious, therefore, you need to applaud every little step in the right direction.

The anorexic child will probably deny they have a problem and tell you to "leave them alone." **Do not give in that easy. Do not leave the child alone unless he/she is completely stabilized.** Seek medical advice and psychiatric treatment.

This disorder can cause extreme behavior when accompanied by depression. It can lead to severe depression and even suicide. **Again, until you are positive your child is stable, do not leave her/him alone.** Even going to the bathroom, showering will require your careful supervision. A child needs you to watch over them during all phases of treatment, especially when re-entering home life following a hospitalization. This transition is very crucial, because the anorexic will need careful monitoring so that he/she does not relapse.

Please realize that the relapse rate for eating disorders is very high and it may take several years to completely recover from an eating disorder.

The anorexic child needs constant assistance in order to beat the disorder. When the doctor gives your child a goal weight and a diet plan, you need to stick with that plan no matter what. You need to prepare all meals as instructed and make sure your child is not hiding food or using other methods to "cheat the system."

I think, if the parent is strict, yet loving and supportive, the eating plan/weight gain will go smoother.

Parents can also help their anorexic child by finding out what they think and exploring their self-talk. You need to help your anorexic child change their own self-talk. Examples of anorexic vs. healthy self-talk are as follows…

Anorexic (Unhealthy) Self-Talk
Needs To Be Changed To Healthy Self-Talk

Anorexic Self-Talk: I don't have a problem, I don't need help.
Healthy Self-Talk: I have a serious eating disorder. I need to seek treatment from doctors and therapists in order to treat and to overcome this disorder.

Anorexic Self-Talk: I am fat.
Healthy Self-Talk: I feel bloated because I am not eating right. If I eat a healthy diet including six small meals a day, then I won't feel bloated.

Anorexic Self-Talk: I want to control my body and my food intake.
Healthy Self-Talk: I want to be healthy and manage this disorder so that I may run, bike, and play sports. If I am healthy, I will have strong muscles and bones.

Anorexic Self-Talk: I want to be thin.
Healthy Self-Talk: I want to be muscular and strong. I want to be in good physical shape and excel in the sport of my choice.

Anorexic Self-Talk: Being really skinny and thin is good. I like to be skinny.

Healthy Self-Talk: Being too thin can lead to a heart attack and death. Also, being too thin over a long period time, can cause a loss of periods in women and lead to early onset of osteoporosis. It can also cause severe problems with my liver and kidneys. I need to be healthy. My body needs good fuel in order to be healthy.

Anorexic Self-Talk: I am bad, I don't deserve to be healthy

Healthy Self-Talk: I am good. I deserve to treat myself and pamper myself. My body needs me to feed it with good food.

Anorexic Self-Talk: I am scared to gain weight

Healthy Self-Talk: I am scared to die of anorexia. I need to seek advice and trust the professionals who are treating me.

Anorexic Self-Talk: I am scared to eat a variety of foods. I will only eat a few foods.

Healthy Self-Talk: I need to eat a wide variety of foods daily so that my body gets the nutrients it deserves.

Anorexic Self-Talk: Everyone is trying to fatten me up

Healthy Self-Talk: Everyone loves me and is trying to help me overcome this serious disorder, so that I may live a normal healthy and happy life.

As a parent, you need to understand what you're child is thinking. **The thoughts of anorexic patients can be very self-destructive.** Of all the psychiatric disorders, anorexia has the highest rate of death. More than 10 percent of anorexics will die from complications due to the disorder.

You need to open up the lines of communication with your child. Try to understand his/her "rationalizations". For example, an anorexic patient may think he/she is fat, but in reality be twenty pounds below a normal weight. You need to really listen to your child's explanation of why they think they are fat. You will need to re-rationalize your child, so that they see in reality, they are not fat at all and in fact, need to gain weight.

One method that may work, is to take a picture or a video of your child in their bathing suit, both front and backsides. Show your child the picture or video and ask if they think this person looks healthy. Sometimes, this may be an eye-opening experience for the patient. It may help your child see how horribly skinny they really are.

Please make every effort to re-program your child to believe in healthy eating patterns and healthy weights. This will take considerable effort on your part, because anorexia is a very stubborn disorder. You will need to really work hard to beat this disorder.

I think the hardest part is to make your child realize that he/she really has to be a healthy weight in order to lead a normal and productive life. Tell your child "you can't cheat your body" because your body rebels when it doesn't get enough nutrients.

Use analogies. Compare your child's body to a car. Explain in simple terms, how a car cannot run without fuel, your body cannot run without adequate nutrition.

Help your child develop a healthy self-image. Most anorexics do not have a very good self-image. They think they are fat and unattractive - the idea of a before and after makeover may appeal to many young girls. As a parent, you may make a deal with your child, if they maintain a healthy weight, they will win a special makeover session - makeup, hair and clothes included. Kids love the idea of a makeover and want to look attractive. New clothes, new wardrobe, new makeup, new hairstyle, can help improve the self-image of a recently recovered patient. They will be surprised how much more attention they may receive from looking healthy and cute - rather than from looking skinny.

Another way to create a healthy self-image is to find out what your child really enjoys and help them develop that special talent. For example, maybe your daughter loves horses and would enjoy taking care of a horse on a farm. This allows the child to develop and enjoy new interests which foster good self-esteem.

Parents, please educate yourself about eating disorders. It is important to realize the widespread use of diets in young girls often leads to eating disorders.

Here a few other ways to help your child:

- Focus your child on creative endeavors that allow them to feel purposeful and productive, for example - art, writing, music, etc. Focus on their skills rather than their appearance.

- Be a good role model, eat healthy foods and exercise daily. You are the child's hero. Be a good role model. Children watch what you "do" more than what you "say". Be a good role model. Provide a consistent, positive example for your child.

- Encourage self-empowerment. Encourage them to take control and manage their disorder.

- Offer your child a choice of foods, for example a banana or a fruit snack. Allow the child to have some control over their dietary intake.

- Realize that anorexia is a problem that cannot be solved by you alone. This is not because you are a "bad" parent, but simply because anorexics need a larger support network in order to become healthy - a team of psychiatrists, doctors, nutritionists and therapists are often required.

- Pay special attention to the siblings of your anorexic child. They need your love and attention during this difficult period. In your quest to solve your child's disorder, do not ignore your other children. Create special times in your day to talk, read, play and love them.

- Set up times to play a one on one sport with your child, for example tennis. Always reward success. Focus on the improvements they make in the sport. Enjoy your special times with them.

- Have your child enter into a team sport in which there are healthy peers (like soccer or softball for example). Some team sports are more likely to emphasize the body shape - like dance or gymnastics. Please, avoid entering your child into these sports if they have an eating disorder.

- Be aware of your child's use of the internet. There are some anorexic websites called pro-anna websites. These websites are written by girls that have severe anorexia and support anorexic behaviors. **These websites could have a very negative influence on your child. Please monitor your child's use of the computer.**

- Tell your child how much you love them. Hug and kiss them goodnight. Tell them a story or talk to them every night before they go to bed. When children are relaxed before bedtime, it is an excellent opportunity to connect and review the day with your child. Find out how their day really went. Ask them lots of questions.

• Realize that there are times when you yourself may need support. Talk to friends and family members about your feelings. Seek out a support group if needed. Some hospitals and clinics provide support groups for friends and family of eating disorders patients. Remember, eating disorders can be very stressful for you as the parent. Make sure you take good care of yourself.

• Try to create peace in your home. Make it a wonderful place for your children to live.

CONCLUSION

In conclusion, anorexia is a very serious eating disorder. Without treatment it can lead to serious complications including death.

Fortunately, today, there are many specialists available to help treat eating disorder patients. I know from personal experience, it is possible to really "recover" and lead a normal life. With the advent of new treatments and medicines, more anorexics are reaching a full recovery than in the past.

I think the key to solving the anorexia, may begin with prevention. If parents, teachers and school counselors are more aware of the signs and symptoms of eating disorders, they can spot the disorder before it becomes a full-blown crisis.

ABOUT THE AUTHOR

Lynn Johnson has Bachelors degree in Psychology from the University of Wisconsin Madison and a Masters Degree from Marquette University - Milwaukee Wisconsin. She graduated with honors and was on the Deans List for 2 years. She also had a full tuition scholarship and research assistantship at Marquette University.

HELP YOURSELF

Academy for Eating Disorders
Montefiore Medical School- Adolescent Medicine
111 E. 210th Street
Bronx, NE 10467
(718) 920-6782

American Anorexia/Bulimia Association
293 Central Park West, Suite #1-R
New York, NY 10024
(212) 501-8351

International Association of Eating Disorder Professionals
123 NW 13th Street #206
Boca Raton, FL 33432
(800) 800-8126